Keto For Foodies

The Ultimate Low-Carb Cookbook

Maria J. Marks

Keto For Foodies

Legal Notice

Copyright (c) 2019 Maria J. Marks

All rights are reserved. No portion of this book may be reproduced or duplicated using any form whether mechanical, electronic, or otherwise. No portion of this book may be transmitted, stored in a retrieval database, or otherwise made available in any manner whether public or private unless specific permission is granted by the publisher.

This book does not offer advice, but merely provides information. The author offers no advice whether medical, financial, legal, or otherwise, nor does the author encourage any person to pursue any specific course of action discussed in this book. This book is not a substitute for professional advice. The reader accepts complete and sole responsibility for the manner in which this book and its contents are used. The publisher and the author

Keto For Foodies

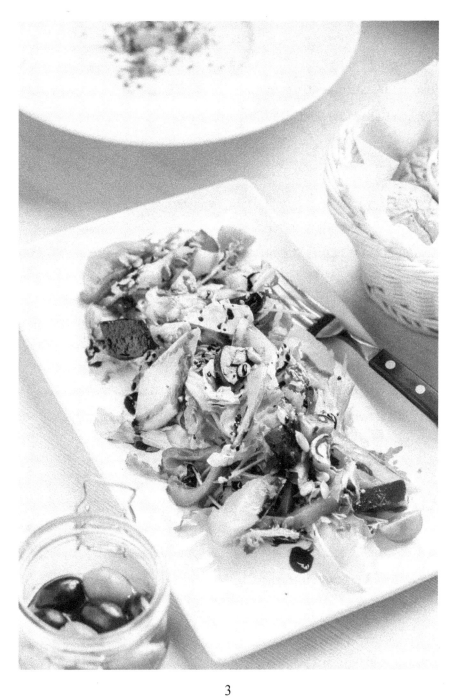

Table of Contents

Chorizo and Peppers.. 8

;Bacon Cheeseburger Casserole 11

Chicken Bacon Chowder 14

Carne Asada... 18

Poached Salmon 20

Ham Soup 22

Creamy Tuscan Garlic Chicken 27

Coconut Cilantro Curry Shrimp.. 30

Pork Chile Verde.. 32

Zuppa Toscana Soup.. 35

Curried Chicken Tacos 37

Spicy Barbecue Shrimp 40

Cabbage Roll Soup... 42

Beef Brisket with Onions 46

Chicken Taco Soup... 49

Soy-Ginger Braised Squid 51

Lamb Barbacoa 54

Reuben Soup 57

Jerk Chicken... 59

Green Beans & Chicken Thighs... 62

Tuna Salpicao... 65

Spicy Pork 66

Sausage and Peppers... 68

Keto For Foodies

Chicken with Bacon Gravy 71

Sausage & Shrimp Gumbo 74

Roast Chicken 77

Bolognese 80

Balsamic Pork Tenderloin 82

Beef and Cheese Stuffed Tomatoes 84

Keto For Foodies

Keto For Foodies

Chorizo and Peppers

Serves: 8 / Preparation time: 5 minutes / Cooking time: 10 hours

2 pounds pasture-raised chorizo sausage, casings removed and crumbled

2 medium green bell peppers, seeded and chopped

2 medium white onion, peeled and chopped

2 tablespoons minced garlic

1 ½ tablespoon avocado oil

6-ounce tomato paste, unsweetened

1 cup water

1 cup red wine

• Place sausage in a 6-quart slow cooker, crumble it, then add

remaining ingredients and stir until combined.

• Plug in the slow cooker, shut with lid and cook for 8 hours at low heat setting or until cooked through.

• Then uncover slow cooker and cook more for 2 hours or until some of

the cooking liquid evaporates.

• Serve straightaway.

One Serving: Net Carbs: 6g; Calories: 370; Total Fat: 25g; Sat. Fat: 2.4g;

Protein: 29g; Carbs: 8g; Fiber: 2g; Sugar: 2.4g Percentage of Calories:

Total Fat: 60%; Protein: 31%; Carbs: 9%

Keto For Foodies

;Bacon Cheeseburger Casserole

Serves: 10 / Preparation time: 5 minutes / Cooking time: 4 hours and 10

minutes

2 pounds ground beef, grass-fed

1/2 pound bacon, cooked and crumbled, divided

1/2 of medium white onion, peeled and sliced

½ teaspoon garlic salt

½ teaspoon salt

½ teaspoon ground black pepper

1 tablespoon avocado oil

2 cups grated cheddar cheese

10.5-ounce cheddar cheese soup

10.5 ounce cream of mushroom soup

● Place a large skillet pan over medium heat, add oil and when hot, add

beef and season with garlic salt, salt, and black pepper.

- Cook for 5 to 7 minutes or until nicely golden brown, then drain fats

from beef and transfer to a greased 6-quarts slow cooker.

- Add all soups and bacon, reversing 2 pieces, stir well, then spread

evenly and top with onion, cheese and remaining bacon at the end.

- Plug in the slow cooker, shut with lid and cook for 4 hours at low heat

setting or until cooked.

- Serve straightaway.

One Serving: Net Carbs: 4g; Calories: 451; Total Fat:

31.6g; Sat. Fat: 16.9g; Protein: 36g; Carbs: 5.6g; Fiber:

1.6g;

Sugar: 1.3g Percentage of Calories: Total Fat: 63%;

Protein: 32%; Carbs: 5%;

Keto For Foodies

Chicken Bacon Chowder

Serves: 6 / Preparation time: 5 minutes / Cooking time: 9 hours and 5

minutes

1 pound pasture-raised chicken breast, skinless

1 pound bacon

6-ounce Cremini mushrooms

2 celery, diced

1 medium white onion, peeled and diced

2 teaspoons minced garlic

1 teaspoon garlic powder

1 teaspoon salt

1 teaspoon ground black pepper

1 teaspoon dried thyme

2 tablespoons avocado oil

2 tablespoons unsalted butter

2 cups chicken stock

8-ounce cream cheese, cubed

1 cup heavy cream

- Plug in a 6-quart slow cooker and let preheat at low heat setting.

- Then add mushrooms, celery, onion, garlic, salt, black pepper, butter,

and 1 cup stock and stir until mixed.

- Shut with lid and cook for 1 hour at low heat setting.

- Place a large skillet pan over medium-high heat, add oil and when

hot, add oil and when hot, add chicken and cook for 5 minutes or

until seared on all sides.

- Transfer seared chicken to a plate, deglaze the pan with remaining

stock and stir well to remove browned bits stuck on the bottom of the

pan and then add to slow cooker when vegetables are cooked.

- Add remaining ingredients to cooked vegetables, stir well until cream

cheese is mixed.

- Cut chicken into cubes, add to slow cooker along with bacon and stir

until mixed.- Shut with lid and cook for 6 to 8 hours at low heat setting or until

cooked through.

- Serve straightaway.

One Serving: Net Carbs: 5.5g; Calories: 879.3; Total Fat: 66.4g; Sat. Fat:

30g; Protein: 59.3g; Carbs: 11g; Fiber: 5.5g; Sugar: 6.5g Percentage of

Calories: Total Fat: 68%; Protein: 27%; Carbs: 5%;

Keto For Foodies

Carne Asada

Serves: 8 / Preparation time: 5 minutes / Cooking time: 8 hours

2 pounds grass-fed steak

2 chipotle peppers in adobo sauce

2 teaspoons minced garlic

1/2 teaspoon sea salt

1/2 teaspoon paprika

1/2 teaspoon ground cumin

1 teaspoon fish sauce, unsweetened

1 tablespoon avocado oil

1/2 cup orange juice

1 lime, juiced

1/4 cup chopped fresh cilantro

Diced avocado for topping

Sour cream for topping

8 large lettuce leaves

• Prepare sauce and for this, place all the ingredients in a food processor, except for steak and toppings, and pulse until smooth, set

aside until required.

● Place a large skillet over medium heat, grease with avocado oil, add

steaks in a single layer and cook for 5 minutes per side or until

brown.

● Plug in the slow cooker, place steaks into it, then top with sauce and

shut with lid.

● Cook for 8 hours at low heat setting or until cooked through.

● When done, shred steaks with two forks and serve as a lettuce wrap

topped with avocado and sour cream.

One Serving: Net Carbs: 5.9g; Calories: 408; Total Fat: 27.2g; Sat. Fat:

11.3g; Protein: 33.6g; Carbs: 7.2g; Fiber: 1.3g; Sugar: 4g Percentage of

Calories: Total Fat: 60%; Protein: 33%; Carbs: 7%;

Poached Salmon

Serves: 4 / Preparation time: 5 minutes / Cooking time: 3

hours and 35

minutes

4 steaks of wild-caught salmon

1 medium white onion, peeled and sliced

2 teaspoons minced garlic

1/2 teaspoon salt

1/8 teaspoon ground white pepper

1/2 teaspoon dried dill weed

2 tablespoons avocado oil

2 tablespoons unsalted butter

2 tablespoons lemon juice

1 cup water

- Place butter in a 4-quart slow cooker, then add salmon and drizzle

with oil.

- Place remaining ingredients in a medium saucepan, stir until mixed

and bring the mixture to boil over high heat.

- Then pour this mixture all over salmon and shut with lid.

- Plug in the slow cooker and cook salmon for 3 hours and 30 minutes

at low heat setting or until salmon is tender.

- Serve straightaway.

One Serving: Net Carbs: 2.8g; Calories: 310; Total Fat: 20g; Sat. Fat: 4.8g;

Protein: 30.2g; Carbs: 3.1g; Fiber: 0.3g; Sugar: 1.2g Percentage of

Calories: Total Fat: 57%; Protein: 39%; Carbs: 4%;

Ham Soup

Serves: 6 / Preparation time: 5 minutes / Cooking time: 4 hours

2 pounds pasture-raised smoked ham hock

4 cups cauliflower florets

2 bay leaves

¼ teaspoon nutmeg

3 cups bone broth

• Place cauliflower florets in a 6-quarts slow cooker, add remaining

ingredients and pour in water until all the ingredients are just

submerged.

• Plug in the slow cooker, then shut with lid and cook for 4 hours at high

heat setting or until cauliflower florets are very tender.

• Transfer ham to a bowl, shred with two forms and discard bone and

fat pieces.

• Puree cauliflower in the slow cooker with a stick blender for 1 to 2

minutes or until smooth, return shredded ham and stir until well

combined.

• Taste soup to adjust seasoning and serve.

One Serving: Net Carbs: 3g; Calories: 349; Total Fat: 23g; Sat. Fat: 10g;

Protein: 34g; Carbs: 5g; Fiber: 2g; Sugar: 2g Percentage of Calories: Total

Fat: 58%; Protein: 37%; Carbs: 5%;Beef Teriyaki Lettuce Cups

Serves: 5 / Preparation time: 5 minutes / Cooking time: 9 hours and 30

minutes

2 pounds grass-fed beef roast, halved lengthwise.

4 green onions, chopped

1 small white onion, peeled and diced

1 ½ teaspoon minced garlic

1 teaspoon grated ginger

4 teaspoons swerve sweetener

2 tablespoons arrowroot

1/2 cup soy sauce

1/3 cup apple cider vinegar

1 tablespoon avocado oil

1/3 cup water

Sesame seeds for garnishing

12 lettuce cups

• Whisk together white onion, garlic, ginger, sweetener, soy sauce,

vinegar, and oil in a small bowl and whisk well until combined.

• Place beef into a 6-quart slow cooker, pour in prepared mixture and

shut with lid.

• Plug in the slow cooker and cook for 8 to 9 hours at low heat setting

or 6 to 7 hours at high heat setting or until beef is very tender.

• When done, transfer beef to a cutting board and let rest.

• In the meantime, stir together arrowroot and water until combined,

add to sauce in the slow cooker and cook at high heat setting for 20

to 30 minutes or until thickened to desired consistency.

• Shred beef with two forms, return to thickened sauce and toss until coated.

- Garnish beef with sesame seeds and green onion and serve in

lettuce cups.One Serving: Net Carbs: 2g; Calories: 526; Total Fat: 32.8g; Sat. Fat:

17.2g; Protein: 52.6g; Carbs: 5.3g; Fiber: 3.3g; Sugar: 1.3g Percentage of

Calories: Total Fat: 56%; Protein: 40%; Carbs: 4%;

Creamy Tuscan Garlic Chicken

Serves: 4 / Preparation time: 5 minutes / Cooking time: 8 hours and 10

minutes

4 large pasture-raised chicken breast, each about 6 ounce

1/2 cup sun-dried tomatoes, chopped

2 cup spinach, chopped

3 teaspoons minced garlic

1 ½ teaspoon sea salt

1 teaspoon ground black pepper

1 tablespoon Italian seasoning

1 tablespoon avocado oil

1 cup heavy cream

1/3 cup chicken broth

3/4 cup grated parmesan cheese

• Place a medium saucepan over medium heat, add oil and when hot,

add garlic and cook for 1 minute or until fragrant.

• Whisk in cream and broth, bring the mixture to simmer, then reduce

heat to a low level and simmer more for 10 minutes or until sauce

thickens enough to coat back of the spoon.

• In the meantime, place chicken in a 6-quarts slow cooker.

• When the sauce is ready, stir in cheese until smooth and then pour

this sauce over chicken.

• Plug in the slow cooker and cook for 6 to 8 hours at low

heat setting

or 3 to 4 hours at high heat setting or until cooked through.

• When done, transfer chicken to a serving plate and set aside.

• Add spinach to sauce in the slow cooker and cook for 3 to 5 minutes

or until spinach leaves wilt.

• Then chicken to slow cooker, spoon sauce over chicken, then top with

tomatoes and serve.One Serving: Net Carbs: 4g; Calories: 531; Total Fat: 35g; Sat. Fat: 11.7g;

Protein: 45g; Carbs: 9g; Fiber: 5g; Sugar: 1g Percentage of Calories: Total

Fat: 60%; Protein: 33%; Carbs: 7%;

Coconut Cilantro Curry Shrimp

Serves: 4 / Preparation time: 5 minutes / Cooking time: 2 hours and 30

minutes

1 pound wild-caught shrimp, peeled and deveined

2 ½ teaspoon lemon garlic seasoning

2 tablespoons red curry paste

4 tablespoons chopped cilantro

30 ounces coconut milk, unsweetened

16 ounces water

- Whisk together all the ingredients except for shrimps and

2

tablespoons cilantro and add to a 4-quart slow cooker.

● Plug in the slow cooker, shut with lid and cook for 2 hours at high heat

setting or 4 hours at low heat setting.

● Then add shrimps, toss until evenly coated and cook for 20 to 30

minutes at high heat settings or until shrimps are pink.

● Garnish shrimps with remaining cilantro and serve.

One Serving: Net Carbs: 1.9g; Calories: 160.7; Total Fat: 8.2g; Sat. Fat:

8.1g; Protein: 19.3g; Carbs: 2.4g; Fiber: 0.5g; Sugar: 1.4g Percentage of

Calories: Total Fat: 46%; Protein: 48%; Carbs: 6%;

Pork Chile Verde

Serves: 6 / Preparation time: 5 minutes / Cooking time: 7 hours and 5

minutes

2 pounds pasture-raised pork shoulder, cut into 6 pieces

1 teaspoon sea salt

½ teaspoon ground black pepper

1 ½ tablespoon avocado oil

1 ½ cup salsa verde

1 cup chicken broth

• Season pork with salt and black pepper.

• Place a large skillet pan over medium heat, add oil and when hot, add

seasoned pork pieces.

- Cook pork for 3 to 4 minutes per side or until browned and then

transfer to a 6-quart slow cooker.

- Whisk together salsa and chicken broth and pour over pork pieces.

- Plug in the slow cooker, then shut with lid and cook for 6 to 7 hours at

low heat setting or until pork is very tender.

- When done, shred pork with two forks and stir until combined. ·

One Serving: Net Carbs: 4g; Calories: 342; Total Fat: 22g; Sat. Fat: 12g;

Protein: 32g; Carbs: 6g; Fiber: 2g; Sugar: 4g Percentage of Calories: Total

Fat: 58%; Protein: 36%; Carbs: 6%;

Keto For Foodies

Zuppa Toscana Soup

Serves: 10 / Preparation time: 5 minutes / Cooking time: 8 hours and 10

minutes

1 pound ground Italian sausage, grass-fed

1 large cauliflower head, cut into small florets

3 cups chopped kale

½ cup diced white onion

1 ½ teaspoon minced garlic

1 teaspoon salt

½ teaspoon ground black pepper

¼ teaspoon crushed red pepper flakes

1 tablespoon avocado oil

36 ounces chicken stock

½ cup heavy cream

● Place a large skillet pan over medium heat, add sausage and cook for

7 to 10 minutes or until nicely brown.

- Drain fat from pan and transfer sausage to a 6-quart slow cooker.

- Add oil into the skillet and when hot, add onion and cook for 3 to 4

minutes or until beginning to soften.

- Transfer onions to the slow cooker cooked, along with remaining

ingredients except for heavy cream and stir until mixed.

- Plug in the slow cooker, then shut with lid and cook for 8 hours at low

heat setting or 4 hours at high heat setting until cooked through.

- When done, stir in heavy cream and serve immediately.

One Serving: Net Carbs: 3g; Calories: 255; Total Fat: 19g; Sat. Fat: 7g;

Protein: 14g; Carbs: 7g; Fiber: 4g; Sugar: 3g Percentage of Calories: Total

Fat: 68%; Protein: 22%; Carbs: 10%;

Curried Chicken Tacos

Serves: 8 / Preparation time: 5 minutes / Cooking time: 8 hours

For Curried Chicken:

2 pounds skinless pasture-raised chicken breasts

15-ounce diced tomatoes

3 chiles de Arbol, chopped

1/2 of medium white onion, chopped

2 teaspoon grated ginger

2 teaspoons minced garlic

1 teaspoon salt

1 1/2 teaspoons ground turmeric

2 teaspoons ground cumin

1 tablespoon ground coriander

1/4 teaspoon cinnamon

1/4 teaspoon ground cardamom

2-star anise

1/2 cup chicken stock

For Avocado Cream:

1 large avocado, pitted

1/3 cup chopped cilantro

2 teaspoons onion powder

1/2 teaspoon salt

1 1/2 teaspoons red chili powder

5 tablespoons yogurt, high-fat

1 1/2 tablespoons lemon juice

For Taco:

1/2 of a small head of red cabbage, sliced

8 large leaves of collard greens

1 large red pepper, sliced

2 cups sour cream

• Place all the ingredients, except for star anise and stock in a 6-quart

slow cooker and toss until just mixed.

• Then pour in chicken stock, add star anise and shut with lid.

• Plug in the slow cooker and cook for 7 to 8 hours at low heat setting

or 4 to5 hours at high heat setting.• In the meantime, prepare avocado cream and for this, place all the

ingredients for avocado cream in a food processor and pulse for 1 to

2 minutes or until smooth, set aside until required.

- Trim tough stem from collard greens, rinse well, pat dry and set aside

until required.

- When chicken is cooked, shred with two forks and toss until coated

with sauce.

- Assemble tacos and for this, arrange collard greens on clean working

space, then top with chicken, cabbage, pepper, avocado cream and

sour cream in the end.

- Serve straightaway.

One Serving: Net Carbs: 6.4g; Calories: 371.25; Total Fat: 19g; Sat. Fat:

8g; Protein: 41g; Carbs: 9g; Fiber: 2.6g; Sugar: 5.5g Percentage of

Calories: Total Fat: 46%; Protein: 44%; Carbs: 10%;

Spicy Barbecue Shrimp

Serves: 6 / Preparation time: 5 minutes / Cooking time: 1 hour and 30 minutes

1 1/2 pounds large wild-caught shrimp, unpeeled

1 green onion, chopped

1 teaspoon minced garlic

1 ½ teaspoon salt

¾ teaspoon ground black pepper

1 teaspoon Cajun seasoning

1 tablespoon hot pepper sauce

¼ cup Worcestershire Sauce

1 lemon, juiced

2 tablespoons avocado oil

1/2 cup unsalted butter, chopped

• Place all the ingredients except for shrimps in a 6-quart slow cooker

and whisk until mixed.

• Plug in the slow cooker, then shut with lid and cook for 30 minutes at

high heat setting.

• Then take out ½ cup of this sauce and reserve.

- Add shrimps to slow cooker.

One Serving: Net Carbs: 2.4g; Calories: 321; Total Fat: 21.4g; Sat. Fat:

10.6g; Protein: 27.3g; Carbs: 4.8g; Fiber: 2.4g; Sugar: 1.2g Percentage of

Calories: Total Fat: 60%; Protein: 34%; Carbs: 6%;

Cabbage Roll Soup

Serves: 9 / Preparation time: 5 minutes / Cooking time: 6 hours and 10

minutes

2 pounds ground pork, pasture-raised

2 cups cauliflower rice

8 cups sliced cabbage

1/2 cup chopped white onion

1/2 cup chopped shallots

1 teaspoon minced garlic

1 teaspoon salt

1 teaspoon ground black pepper

1 teaspoon dried parsley

1/2 teaspoon dried oregano

2 tablespoons avocado oil

16 ounces marinara sauce, sugar-free and organic

5 cups beef broth

• Place a medium skillet pan over medium-high heat, add oil and when

hot, add onion and shallots and cook for 5 minutes or until softened.

• Add garlic, cook for 30 seconds or until fragrant, then add pork and

cook for 5 to 7 minutes or until nicely browned.

• Season with salt, black pepper, parsley, and oregano, pour in

marinara sauce and stir well.

• Then add cauliflower rice, stir until evenly coated and transfer the

mixture into a 6-quart slow cooker.

- Plug in the slow cooker, pour in beef broth, then add cabbage and stir

until combined.

- Shut with lid and cook for 6 hours at low heat setting or 3 hours at

high setting.

- Serve straightaway. One Serving: Net Carbs: 6g; Calories: 346; Total Fat: 26 g; Sat. Fat: 8g;

Protein: 20g; Carbs: 8g; Fiber: 2g; Sugar: 3g Percentage of Calories: Total

Fat: 68%; Protein: 23%; Carbs: 9%;

Keto For Foodies

Beef Brisket with Onions

Serves: 6 / Preparation time: 5 minutes / Cooking time: 8 hours and 20

minutes

3 1/2 pounds beef brisket, grass-fed

2 large onion, sliced into half moons

3 teaspoons minced garlic

1 teaspoon salt

½ ground black pepper

4 tablespoons avocado oil, divided

2 tablespoons Worcestershire sauce

1 tablespoon soy sauce

2 cups beef broth

- Place a large skillet pan over medium heat, add 2

tablespoons oil and

when hot, add onions and cook for 20 minutes or until lightly

caramelized.

- In the meantime, season brisket with salt and black pepper.

- Place another skillet pan over medium-high heat, then add remaining

oil and seasoned brisket and cook for 5 to 7 minutes or until golden

brown.

- Transfer brisket to 6-quart slow cooker, fat-side up, and sprinkle with

garlic.

- When onions are caramelized, arrange them around brisket.

- Whisk together Worcestershire sauce, soy sauce, and broth until

combined, then pour in the slow cooker and shut with lid.

- Plug in the slow cooker and cook for 6 to 8 hours at low heat setting or until cooked through.

- When done, let brisket rest for 20 minutes and then shred with two

forks

- Serve shredded brisket with onions. One Serving: Net Carbs: 1.3g; Calories: 246; Total Fat: 19g; Sat. Fat: 6.6g;

Protein: 17g; Carbs: 2g; Fiber: 0.7g; Sugar: 3g Percentage of Calories:

Total Fat: 70%; Protein: 27%; Carbs: 3%;

Chicken Taco Soup

Serves: 8 / Preparation time: 5 minutes / Cooking time: 4 hours and 10

minutes

2 pounds pasture-raised ground chicken

2 tablespoons chopped cilantro

20-ounce Rotel tomatoes

2 tablespoons taco seasoning

2 tablespoons avocado oil

16-ounce cream cheese

1/2 cup grated cheddar cheese and more for garnishing

4 cup chicken broth

• Place a large skillet pan over medium heat, add oil and when hot, add

beef and cook for 7 to 10 minutes or until cooked and nicely golden

brown.

• In the meantime, place tomatoes, seasoning and cream cheese in a

6-quart slow cooker and plug it in.

- When beef is done, drain fat from pan and transfer beef to slow

cooker.

- Stir until combined, then pour in broth, add cheese and shut with lid.

- Cook for 4 hours at low heat setting or 2 hours at high heat setting or

until cooked through.

- Garnish with more cheese and serve.

One Serving: Net Carbs: 3.8g; Calories: 585.5; Total Fat: 45.5g; Sat. Fat:

20.6g; Protein: 39.5g; Carbs: 4.4g; Fiber: 0.6g; Sugar: 4g Percentage of

Calories: Total Fat: 70%; Protein: 27%; Carbs: 3%;

Soy-Ginger Braised Squid

Serves: 6 / Preparation time: 5 minutes / Cooking time: 8 hours

18-ounce wild-caught squid, cut into rings

2 scallions, chopped

2 bay leaves

1 tablespoon grated ginger

1 bulb of garlic, peeled and minced

½ cup swerve sweetener

¼ cup soy sauce

¼ cup oyster sauce

¼ cup avocado oil

¼ cup white wine

- Plug in a 6-quart slow cooker, add all the ingredients and stir until

mixed.

- Shut with lid and cook for 8 hours at low heat setting or until cooked

through.

- Serve straightaway.

One Serving: Net Carbs: 3.1g; Calories: 135.2; Total Fat: 9.2g; Sat. Fat:

1.2g; Protein: 9.8g; Carbs: 3.4g; Fiber: 0.3g; Sugar: 1.23g Percentage of

Calories: Total Fat: 61%; Protein: 29%; Carbs: 10%;

Lamb Barbacoa

Serves: 12 / Preparation time: 5 minutes / Cooking time: 8 hours

5 pounds pasture-raised pork shoulder, fat trimmed

2 tablespoons salt

1 teaspoon chipotle powder

2 tablespoons smoked paprika

1 tablespoon ground cumin

1 tablespoon dried oregano

¼ cup dried mustard

1 cup water

- Stir together salt, chipotle powder, paprika, cumin, oregano, and

mustard and rub this mixture generously on all over the pork.

- Place seasoned pork into a 6-quart slow cooker, plug it in, then shut

with lid and cook for 6 hours at high heat setting.

- When done, shred pork with two forks and stir well until coated well.

- Serve straightaway.

One Serving: Net Carbs: 0.7g; Calories: 477; Total Fat: 35.8g; Sat. Fat:

14.8g; Protein: 37.5g; Carbs: 1.2g; Fiber: 0.5g; Sugar: 5g Percentage of

Calories: Total Fat: 68%; Protein: 31%; Carbs: 1%;

Keto For Foodies

Reuben Soup

Serves: 12 / Preparation time: 5 minutes / Cooking time: 7 hours

2 pounds grass-fed corned beef, diced

1 pound sauerkraut

1 medium white onion, peeled and diced

1 ½ teaspoon minced garlic

1 teaspoon coriander seeds

1 teaspoon dill seeds

1/2 teaspoon celery seeds

1 tablespoon mustard seeds

2 tablespoons unsalted butter

8 cups beef broth

2 cups heavy cream

8 ounce shredded Swiss cheese

- Place a medium skillet pan over medium heat, add 1 tablespoon

butter and when it melts, add onion and cook for 5 minutes or until

tender.

- Then add garlic and continue cooking for 1 minute or until fragrant.

- Spoon this mixture into a 6-quart slow cooker, along with remaining

ingredients except for cream and cheese and stir until mixed.

- Plug in the slow cooker, then shut with lid and cook for 7 hours at low

heat setting or 3 ½ hours at high heat setting.

- When 1 hour of the cooking hour is left, stir in cream and cheese and

continue cooking until cooked through.

- Serve straightaway.

One Serving: Net Carbs: 1.9g; Calories: 343; Total Fat: 26.3g; Sat. Fat:

11g; Protein: 23g; Carbs: 3.4g; Fiber: 1.5g; Sugar: 5g Percentage of

Calories: Total Fat: 69%; Protein: 27%; Carbs: 4%;

Jerk Chicken

Serves: 8 / Preparation time: 5 minutes / Cooking time: 6

hours and 15

minutes

4 pounds skin-on pasture-raised chicken pieces

8 scallions, chopped

2 habanero chilies, cored and seeded

1 ½ teaspoon minced garlic

1 tablespoon grated ginger

2 tablespoons swerve sweetener

1 teaspoon salt

1 tablespoon dried thyme

2 teaspoons allspice

1/4 teaspoon cardamom

1/4 cup avocado oil

1 cup sour cream for serving

• Place all the ingredients in a blender, except for chicken and sour

cream, and process until smooth.

• Transfer ½ cup of this mixture in a 4-quart slow cooker, add chicken and turn to coat with the mixture.

- Plug in the slow cooker, shut with lid and cook for 4 to 6 hours at low

heat setting or until cooked through.

- In the meantime, switch on the broiler, place an oven rack about 10-

inch away from the heating source and let preheat.

- Take a sheet pan, line with aluminum foil, then grease with oil and

place cooked chicken on it.

- Place sheet pan into the oven and broil for 10 to 15 minutes per side

or until crispy.

- Serve with sour cream.

One Serving: Net Carbs: 1.1g; Calories: 666; Total Fat: 42.2g; Sat. Fat:

18.9g; Protein: 70g; Carbs: 1.6g; Fiber: 0.5g; Sugar: 1.5g Percentage of

Calories: Total Fat: 57%; Protein: 42%; Carbs: 1%;

Green Beans & Chicken Thighs

Serves: 4 / Preparation time: 5 minutes / Cooking time: 8 hours

4 skin-on pasture-raised chicken thighs

1 pound green beans, trimmed

2 large tomatoes, diced

1 medium white onion, peeled and diced

1 teaspoon minced garlic

2 teaspoons salt and more for seasoning chicken

1 teaspoon ground black pepper and more for seasoning

chicken

1/4 cup fresh chopped dill

6 tablespoons avocado oil, divided

1 lemon, juiced

1 cup chicken broth

1 cup sour cream

- Place green beans in a 6-quarts slow cooker, add remaining

ingredients except for 3 tablespoons oil, chicken and sour cream and

stir until mixed.

- Plug in slow cooker, top green beans with chicken, drizzle with oil,

season with salt and black pepper and shut with lid.

- Cook for 8 hours at low heat setting or for 4 hours at high heat setting

or until chicken is cooked through.

- Serve with sour cream.

One Serving: Net Carbs: 7g; Calories: 622; Total Fat: 46.3g; Sat. Fat:

12.3g; Protein: 35.7g; Carbs: 15.5g; Fiber: 8.5g; Sugar: 9.3g Percentage of

Calories: Total Fat: 67%; Protein: 23%; Carbs: 10%;

Tuna Salpicao

Serves: 3 / Preparation time: 5 minutes / Cooking time: 4 hours and 10

minutes

8 ounce cooked wild-caught tuna, cut into inch cubes

4 jalapeno peppers, chopped

5 red chili, chopped

1 bulb of garlic, peeled and minced

1 teaspoon salt

1 teaspoon ground black pepper

1 cup avocado oil

• Place all the ingredients except for tuna in a 4-quart slow cooker and

stir until mixed.

• Plug in the slow cooker, shut with lid and cook for 4 hours at low heat setting.

- Then add tuna and continue cooking for 10 minutes at high heat

setting.

- Serve straightaway.

One Serving: Net Carbs: 0.8g; Calories: 737.6; Total Fat: 72.1g; Sat. Fat:

8.6g; Protein: 20.2g; Carbs: 1.8g; Fiber: 0.6g; Sugar: 1g Percentage of

Calories: Total Fat: 88%; Protein: 11%; Carbs: 1%;

Spicy Pork

Serves: 6 / Preparation time: 5 minutes / Cooking time: 10 hours

2 pasture-raised pork shoulder, boneless and fat trimmed

½ of jalapeno, deseeded and cored, chopped

6 ounce crushed tomatoes

¼ cup chopped green onion

3 clove of garlic, peeled and sliced in half

1 tablespoon sea salt

½ teaspoon ground black pepper

1 ½ tablespoon paprika, divided

½ tablespoon dried oregano

½ tablespoon ground cumin

2 limes, juiced

2 tablespoons avocado oil

● Place pork in a 6-quart slow cooker, season with salt, black pepper,

paprika, oregano, and cumin until seasoned well.

● Then add remaining ingredients and stir until combined.

● Plug in the slow cooker, shut it with the lid and cook for 8 to 10 hours

at low heat setting or 4 to 5 hours at high heat setting until very

tender.

- Serve straightaway.

One Serving: Net Carbs: 1.2g; Calories: 344.5; Total Fat: 25g; Sat. Fat:

10.7g; Protein: 28.4g; Carbs: 1.7g; Fiber: 0.5g; Sugar: 1.1g Percentage of

Calories: Total Fat: 65%; Protein: 33%; Carbs: 2%;

Sausage and Peppers

Serves: 8 / Preparation time: 5 minutes / Cooking time: 6 hours

2 pounds grass-fed Italian sausage links

4 medium green bell peppers, cored and thinly sliced

28-ounce unsalted crushed tomatoes

2 large white onions, peeled and thinly sliced

3 teaspoons minced garlic

1 tablespoon salt

1 teaspoon Italian Seasoning

1/4 teaspoon dried oregano

1/2 teaspoon crushed red pepper flakes

1 bay leaf

3 tablespoons avocado oil

1/4 cup chilled water

Chopped parsley for serving

Sour cream for topping

- Place all the ingredients except for parsley and cream in a 6-quart

slow cooker and stir until mixed.

- Plug in the slow cooker, shut with lid and cook for 6 hours at low heat

setting or until cooked through.

- When done, garnish with parsley, then top with sour cream and serve.

One Serving: Net Carbs: 6.1g; Calories: 452.5; Total Fat: 34.7g; Sat. Fat:

17g; Protein: 23.7g; Carbs: 11.3g; Fiber: 5.2g; Sugar: 5.2g

Percentage of

Calories: Total Fat: 69%; Protein: 21%; Carbs: 10%;

Chicken with Bacon Gravy

Serves: 5 / Preparation time: 5 minutes / Cooking time: 3 hours and 30

minutes

1 ½ pound skinless pasture-raised chicken breasts

6 slices of bacon, cooked and crumbled

1 teaspoon minced garlic

¼ teaspoon ground black pepper

1 teaspoon dried thyme

3 ½ tablespoons dried chicken gravy mix

4 tablespoons oil

1¼ cup water

1 cup heavy cream

- Place chicken in a 4-quart slow cooker, add bacon and

sprinkle with

garlic, black pepper and garlic and drizzle with oil.

● Whisk together water and chicken gravy mix until smooth and then

pour this mixture over the chicken.

● Plug in the slow cooker, shut with lid and cook for 3 ½ hours at high

heat setting or until chicken is cooked through.

● When done, add cream, then shred chicken with 2 forks and stir until

well combined.

● Serve straightaway.

One Serving: Net Carbs: 1.3g; Calories: 551; Total Fat: 38g; Sat. Fat:

15.3g; Protein: 51g; Carbs: 1.3g; Fiber: 0g; Sugar: 1.5g Percentage of

Calories: Total Fat: 62%; Protein: 37%; Carbs: 1%;

Keto For Foodies

Sausage & Shrimp Gumbo

Serves: 6 / Preparation time: 5 minutes / Cooking time: 4 hours and 35

minutes

¾ pound pasture-raised Smoked sausage, sliced into ½ pieces

1 pound wild-caught shrimp, peeled and deveined

1 medium white onion, peeled and diced

1 medium green bell pepper, diced

14.5 ounce diced tomatoes

1/8 teaspoon ground red pepper

2 teaspoons dried oregano

2 teaspoons dried thyme

¼ cup almond flour

2 tablespoons avocado oil

1¼ cup chicken broth

• Place tomatoes in a 6-quart slow cooker, add broth and stir until

mixed.

• Place a small skillet over high heat, add flour and cook

for 3 to 4

minutes or until nicely browned.

- Then reduce heat to low, stir in oil until smooth and spoon the mixture

into slow cooker.

- Add remaining ingredients except for shrimps and stir well.

- Plug in the slow cooker, shut with lid and cook for 3 hours and 30

minutes at low heat setting.

- Then add shrimps and cook for 1 hour or until done.

- Serve gumbo with cauliflower rice.

One Serving: Net Carbs: 5.21g; Calories: 360.5; Total Fat: 22.8g; Sat. Fat:

6g; Protein: 31.5g; Carbs: 7.21g; Fiber: 2g; Sugar: 4g Percentage of

Calories: Total Fat: 57%; Protein: 35%; Carbs: 8%;

Keto For Foodies

Roast Chicken

Serves: 4 / Preparation time: 5 minutes / Cooking time: 5 hours and 35

minutes

1 medium pasture-raised whole chicken

1 large onion, peeled and cut into thick slices

1 ½ teaspoon salt

1 teaspoon ground black pepper

1 bay leaf

4 tablespoons avocado oil

½ cup boiling water

• Preheat a 6-quart slow cooker over low heat setting.

• Then place spread onion all over the bottom of slow cooker and pour

in boiling water.

• Whisk together salt, black pepper, and oil and brush this mixture all

over the inside and outside of the chicken, and then place bay leaf in

the cavity.

- Place chicken on top onions, shut with lid, cook for 5 hours at low

heat setting and then tip chicken to flow out the liquid present inside

the chicken.

- Continue cooking chicken at high heat setting for 30 minutes and then

broil for 5 to 10 minutes or until its skin is nicely golden brown.

- In the meantime, pass the vegetable mixture in slow cooker through a

sieve and press gently.

- Serve this gravy with chicken.

One Serving: Net Carbs: 5g; Calories: 494; Total Fat: 30g; Sat. Fat: 10g;

Protein: 49g; Carbs: 7g; Fiber: 2g; Sugar: 6g Percentage of Calories: Total

Fat: 55%; Protein: 40%; Carbs: 5%;

Keto For Foodies

Bolognese

Serves: 4 / Preparation time: 5 minutes / Cooking time: 4 hours

1 pound ground beef, grass-fed

14.5 ounce diced tomatoes

1 teaspoon onion powder

1 teaspoon salt

½ teaspoon ground black pepper

1 teaspoon Italian seasoning

3 tablespoons avocado oil

8-ounce tomato sauce

3 bay leaves

• Place a large skillet pan over medium heat, add beef, season with

onion powder and Italian seasoning and cook for 7 to 10 minutes or

until nicely browned.

• Then drain fat from the pan, transfer beef to a 6-quart slow cooker

and add remaining ingredients.

- Plug in the slow cooker, stir all the ingredients until just mix, then shut

with lid and cook for 4 hours at low heat setting or 8 hours at high

heat setting until cooked.

- Serve straightaway.

One Serving: Net Carbs: 4g; Calories: 411.5; Total Fat: 28.8g; Sat. Fat:

17g; Protein: 31.9g; Carbs: 6g; Fiber: 2g; Sugar: 5g Percentage of

Calories: Total Fat: 63%; Protein: 31%; Carbs: 6%;

Balsamic Pork Tenderloin

Serves: 8 / Preparation time: 5 minutes / Cooking time: 6 hours

2 pounds pasture-raised pork tenderloin

2 teaspoons minced garlic

1/2 teaspoon sea salt

1/2 teaspoon red pepper flakes

1 tablespoon Worcestershire sauce

2 tablespoons avocado oil

1/2 cup balsamic vinegar

2 tablespoons coconut aminos

• Grease a 6-quart slow cooker with oil and set aside.

• Sprinkle garlic all over the pork and then place it into the slow cooker.

• Whisk together remaining ingredients, then pour over pork and shut

with lid.

• Plug in the slow cooker and cook pork for 6 hours at low heat setting

or 4 hours at high setting until tender.

- When done, transfer pork to serving plate, pour ½ cup of cooking

liquid over pork and serve.

One Serving: Net Carbs: 0.6g; Calories: 224; Total Fat: 10g; Sat. Fat: 1.6g;

Protein: 33g; Carbs: 0.6g; Fiber: 0g; Sugar: 0.3g Percentage of Calories:

Total Fat: 40%; Protein: 59%; Carbs: 1%;

Beef and Cheese Stuffed Tomatoes

Serves: 4 / Preparation time: 5 minutes / Cooking time: 4 hours

¼ pound ground beef, grass-fed

4 large tomatoes

1 green pepper, chopped

1 stalk of green onion, chopped

½ teaspoon salt

½ teaspoon ground black

½ teaspoon dried parsley

4 tablespoons avocado oil

¾ cup beef broth

6 tablespoons grated Mozzarella cheese

6 tablespoon grated parmesan cheese

• Remove top off from each tomato and then scoop out its pulp with a

small spoon.

• Transfer tomato pulp into a large bowl, add beef, green pepper, onion, salt, and black pepper and stir until combined.

- Spoon this mixture into each tomato, then sprinkle 1 ½ tablespoon of

mozzarella and parmesan cheese on top of each tomato, sprinkle

with parsley and then brush with oil.

- Plug in 4-quarts slow cooker, then pour in beef broth, add stuffed

tomatoes and shut with lid.

- Cook for 2 to 4 hours at high heat setting or until tomatoes are tender.

- Serve straightaway.

One Serving: Net Carbs: 6.5g; Calories: 369; Total Fat: 30.3g; Sat. Fat:

17g; Protein: 15g; Carbs: 9.2g; Fiber: 3.3g; Sugar: 6 Percentage of

Calories: Total Fat: 74%; Protein: 16%; Carbs: 10%;S

CPSIA information can be obtained
at www.ICGtesting.com
Printed in the USA
BVHW090048280421
605722BV00022B/1003